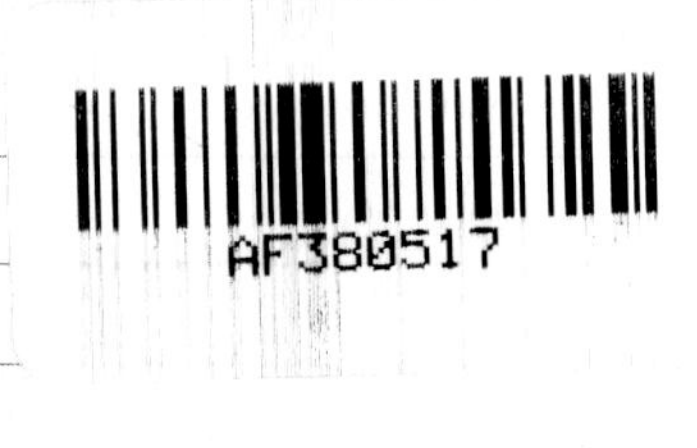

Made in the USA
Monee, IL
07 July 2026

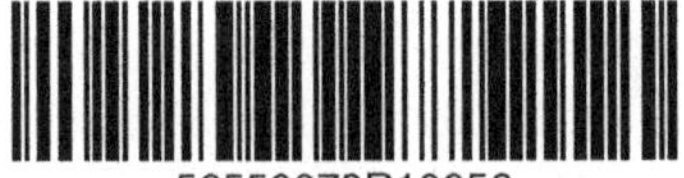

56550079R10056